Working Through the Valley

Valley

A Caregiver's Journey

Robert Jeter

Walking through the Valley
A Caregiver's Journey

Budding Bard Publishing

Copyright © 2002 by Robert Jeter

Editorial Offices: 511 New Kent Place
Cary, NC 27511-7603 USA

Published in the United States of America

Library of Congress
Jeter, Robert
Walking through the valley: A caregiver's journey /
Robert Jeter

ISBN 0-9723206-0-1

Cover and Illustrations by Carl Almblad
Editing and book design by Christena Schafale

In Memory of Ella

Table of Contents

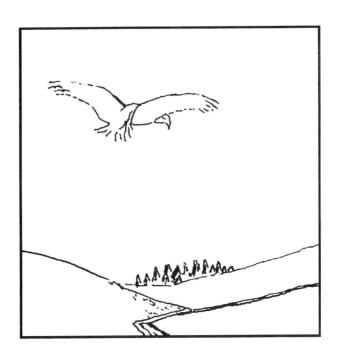

The lone wild bird in lofty flight
Is still with thee nor leaves thy sight
And I am thine, I rest in thee
Great Spirit, come, and rest in me.

The Lone Wild Bird, verse 1
Words by Henry Richard McFadyen.

Preface

Ella and I didn't begin retirement with long-term caregiving as our first choice for living out our days. Rather, like most other seniors, we looked toward our release from the cares of forty-plus years of childrearing and employment – a time when we could enjoy our children (and grandchildren) from afar, being available when needed, but ready to gallivant off to all those places we had dreamed of but never had the opportunity to experience.

For six years, we were able to do much of what we had planned. Then, Ella's lung condition, sarcoidosis, progressed to the point that she required supplemental oxygen and the aid of a pulmonary exercise group, in order to keep the disease process in a relative state of remission. The trips away from Cary/Raleigh dwindled to one every now and then. Thus began the slow, inexorable descent into our respective roles as disabled person and caregiver. My beloved's stroke, suffered on Mother's Day, 1997, signaled the beginning of the final leg of her journey.

The following vignettes from this long trek are a chronicle of our walk through the valley of travail, the moment of Ella's passing, and my long road back up and out of that valley, to once again connect with the land of the living.

Various Pot Pourri articles since 1997 have spotlighted significant events in our lives. These essays have taken a natural progression into the Caregiver Journey essays of 2000 and later. They arose spontaneously out of the need to find meaning in what, at times, seemed totally fractured lives. Our thoughts and emotions cried out for expression, often in the midst of crisis. Nothing less than a written expression of this overflow of long-term grief and emotion would have sufficed.

The first article, "Gone to Sea", reflects our last major trip together, some six months after Ella's stroke.

On Caregiving: Early Stage

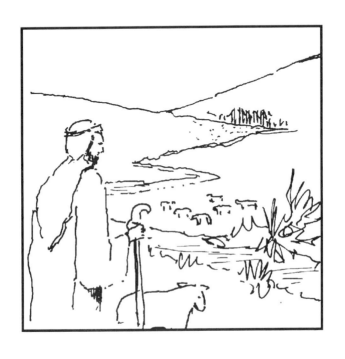

"The Lord is my shepherd,
I shall not want..."
Psalm 23:1
Bible, King James Version

Gone To Sea

December 17, 1997

Ella and I walked into the pulmonary exercise class in early December. Christine spied us and began to whoop it up, "Here come the honeymooners! Here come the honeymooners!" Class members gathered around with questions about our just completed trip. No, we hadn't just gotten hitched. But it had been like the extended honeymoon we never took in 1954. We were just back from a wonderful seven-day cruise through the U.S. Virgin Islands and Nassau, Bahamas — our first in nearly forty-four years of marriage, possibly our only such trip ever.

The Westerdam left Fort Lauderdale on a cloudy Saturday evening. After a day and a half of cruising the warm and relatively calm Atlantic, the skies cleared. Shortly, we landed and walked the narrow streets of Philipsburg, St. Maarten's. Later, we perused the many shops of St. Thomas' Charlotte Amalia, and roamed the streets and shops of Nassau in a warm, misty rain. Like others, we did the tourist thing – shopping for T-shirts, caps, and a gold-mounted amethyst ring. Aboard ship, from the many professional shows, games, activities, photo sessions, shops, casino, et al, Ella and I picked and chose. Our favorites were the evening shows and occasional walk around the Upper Promenade Deck. Mind you, all of this with Ella in a wheelchair and me pushing her. (Our good friend, John Adams, whose enthusiasm led us to make the trip in the first place, spelled me in pushing up and down Nassau's steep hills and through the narrow market district.) All this was highlighted by fabulous food for the body, and friendly co-passengers and staff to warm the heart.

Now, I narrate all this to bring home one relevant point: It's never too late to take that trip of a lifetime, if you really want it, no matter how rough the medical or physical problems may seem. We made up our mind to go, back in mid-September, rather late for planning such an excursion. Our primary concern was to secure 24-hour-a-day supplemental oxygen throughout the trip, from plane liftoff at Raleigh-Durham Airport on Saturday, November 29th, to touchdown again on December 6th. It took constant efforts over a two-month period, to assure that everything would go off without a hitch. But, in the end, oxygen and the equipment to administer it was in place at every point in the flights and along the seaways and shore trips, as needed and planned.

Were we the only medically/physically restricted persons on this cruise? Not by a long shot! We noted several wheelchair passengers in various settings, aboard ship and on shore. Several persons used walkers. And regularly, a crutch-bearer moved alongside us. Ships are not the most handicapped-accessible places; but helpful and courteous staff, and understanding fellow-passengers, by and large, helped keep travel frustrations, on board and in transfer to shore destinations, to a minimum.

So, take heart. With good, persistent planning, YOUR dream vacation may just be possible, too. Bon Voyage!

Hey, Hey! Look What I Found!

May 12, 1999

A few months back, a year and a half into fulltime caregiving – Ella had a stroke in May of 1997 – things began to unravel. I was twenty-five pounds overweight, depressed and beginning to experience increased heart rate and blood pressure. This was despite all the exercise, bowling and other diversionary activities. Here was Mr. Professional Counselor, falling apart like everyone else, when subjected to long-term, constant pressure!

One of Ella's pulmonary class therapists heard my story and immediately scheduled me to see their counseling psychologist. A few sessions with Deb did wonders for both heart rate and blood pressure. But that didn't solve all the problems: I needed long-term support, to clear the air regularly and find out how to handle caregiving problems and stresses. The psychologist was available for bi-weekly, one-on-one counseling for several months. I finally became motivated to lose some weight, as well as find respite from the daily, twenty-four hour grind. First, our daughter offered to take her mother out every Thursday evening. Alice also agreed to keep Ella during my Spring Elderhostel week in the Southern Appalachians. This respite became a Godsend. It allowed me to clear both head **and** emotions, so I could concentrate on other stuff!

Now for the weight challenge! January and February were breakthrough months. Using an unconventional low carbohydrate / high protein diet, I was able to lose twenty pounds in eight weeks. With increased cholesterol levels, I heeded my physician's advice to discontinue the new diet and return to a more normal eating pattern. Within three months, and after that fabulous week in the Appalachians, five pounds returned to my 5' 4" frame. So, I tightened up the diet a little – cut the carbohydrates back a bit. The weight stabilized and headed down slightly. Concurrently, Ella and Alice were doing their Thursday Night thing, and I was free to read, practice bowl, or whatever. It was most relaxing.

Physically, since January, I have continued exercising three times a week, added a once-a-week leg stretching routine with an exercise therapist, and made daily walks mandatory. A month ago, those walks increased to about two miles a day.

What has all this gotten me? Well, I've lost a lot of things, for certain.

First off, the emotional load is far less. Short breaks help me immensely, to relax. Secondly, with stretching and daily walks, back pains are diminished and my heart rate has lowered significantly. Another change is, that with proper eating, nutritional supplements and exercise, my cholesterol levels now fall into the normal range for the first time in years.

You want to know another thing I lost? I no longer carry extra pounds, equivalent to two thirteen-pound bowling balls. Last week I was taking two such balls out of the bag and thinking to myself: "How have I carried this much extra load for ten years, without a heart attack? It makes me tired, just to think about it!"

And, what have I gained? Well, for one thing, I now have a better perspective. I touch base with the psychologist, briefly, every two to four weeks. Ventilate a little. Work on things that bother me. Explore other respite possibilities.

With this, I have less of the feeling that I'm "going it alone". I also have more energy, both physical and emotional. I am more light-hearted. And, I have more flexibility to explore and develop that latent comic and light-hearted aspect that I spoke of a couple of months ago.

What have I found? I've found a physically lighter, more energetic person. I've found a happier, brighter personality. And best of all, I've found support and new friendship with my daughter. Oh yes. Ella and I are much closer, through all of this. That alone is worth it all.

My-O-My! Where Does Time Fly?

July 9, 1999

I've just taken down that big wall calendar, to schedule July's events. So much for good intentions: The first week of the month is already gone, and boy was it a humdinger!

For starters, I forgot that our maid, Debbie, was due in on Monday. Then I forgot she'd be early - a client had cancelled. Well, returning from the Wellness Center, I spotted Debbie gathering her equipment, ready to leave. Oops! I forgot to leave her pay! Frantically, I helped Ella from the car, then bounded into the house as our maid-in-waiting finished packing her van and returned to the house. We greeted "Hello", in sync it seemed, as I quickly slipped into the kitchen and placed an envelope, marked "Debbie", on the counter. That was close! She came up quickly from behind, removed the check, and was out the door. "Bye", we simultaneously intoned.

I'm staring at that calendar. It stares right back at me.

"Whatever happened to all that extra time we were supposed to have when we retired?" I'm now thinking. During the final moments before kicking the traces of my 9:00 to 5:00 grind, how I had drooled over that upcoming free time. FREE TIME! What I wouldn't do with all those gamboling minutes, now skipping

11

over the meadows of retirement!

You guessed it. Anticipation exceeded results. Retirement. After the first six years of retirement "freedom", all I now had was one big hassle, finding time for all those things I had dreamed of. It was the same old stuff as B.R. – Before Retirement. "Now those frisky free minutes and hours are all hooked up to the cart of daily routine, never again to roam," I moan as I peer at that calendar, already half full before I even start. Oh yeah. We did have about six years when we roved the East Coast, going to various timeshares, seeing friends, visiting kith and kin. Since then, it's been something of a drag, if the truth be known. That graphic drill sergeant in front of me tells the tale:

Monday-Wednesday-Friday, 10:30 AM to 1:00 PM, locked in for Ella's Wellness Center Pulmonary Class and my fitness program. Tuesday, I bowl. What about the first and third Thursdays, 2:00 to 4:00 PM? That's when I lead a Cary Senior Center Creative Expression Group. Ella attends that, also. On alternate Fridays, she gets her hair washed or cut; mine goes longer between barberings – six weeks. Saturday is Wash Day. Sunday belongs to the church, after which we eat out.

Let's see now: Forty hours, minimum, set in solid concrete. How can I slip all the "elective" stuff into the crevices of that rapidly filling and hardening mass of events? Things like the third Monday meeting of Carolina Health and Humor Association; my Tuesday course on Psychoanalytic Principles of

Creativity; a Wednesday course on Humor Writing; Reiki Class for Ella on Thursday evenings; and various and sundry special events like the six Raleigh Little Theatre plays this year, my participation in monthly Raleigh News and Observer Community Panel meetings, Saturday work on a Habitat for Humanity house, anniversaries, trips to see the children and grandchildren, etc. Good Grief! I haven't even mentioned grocery shopping, cooking, house and yard upkeep, and other necessaries. I'm certainly in lock step almost every day of every week.

So, where's the time for creating and re-creating: Activities like relaxing, thinking, meditating, imagining; singing, dancing, playing an instrument; and dreaming up and fleshing out comedy routines, monologues, stories and dramas for the written page? Tell me, Calendar, tell me – please do!

As I stare up at that Simon Legree, I now admit that my slavery is self-imposed, ME-made. So I guess it's up to ME to apply the jackhammer to the concrete calendar; or, more appropriately, the eraser to this gosh-awful mish-mash of contrived events.

So, simplify! Do what's needed and leave the rest undone. More realistically, X out a third or fourth of those "elective" events, and substitute for them "down" time; doodling time; playing time. Really. And that's what I recently learned during that week off in the Appalachians. For five days, I walked with Nature, observing wildlife and flora; listened to Indian and Appalachian folk tales; square danced into a pleasant tiredness; feasted on delicious, nourishing country food; and talked, and joked and laughed along with fifty total strangers, who were there doing the same things I did. Hopefully, we all learned that one lesson: SIMPLIFY.

Where does time fly? It flies to where I send it. So, I think I'll call it back, just let it be there. Then, maybe that self-imposed straitjacket will loosen a bit. N-o-w: Back to the wall with you Calendar! You're no match for my eraser!

When One Is Not Enough

March 12, 2000

I should have known better than to think I
had everything under control. Ella's brother,
Tom, was as healthy as they come, for 79.
Then he developed acute leukemia and died
within three months. We were thankful he had
never been seriously ill before, and didn't go
through a long-term and debilitating trauma.
Nevertheless, Ella was deeply despondent at
the sudden loss; and her own chronic
condition, involving 11 years of lung
sarcoidosis and a stroke three years ago,
worsened. She has recovered somewhat, but
very slowly. Me? I'm struggling to return to my
more recent positive outlook.

Which brings me to a critical issue for most
caregivers: going it alone. Can it be done
without help from other folks? Probably, I
think, for a little while. But, in the end,
caregiving for a loved one exacts its price.
Even with weekly respite, compliments of our
daughter Alice, the daily grind has noticeably
sapped my physical energy, and put a damper
on my spirit. To give me a break from 24-hour,
seven day a week responsibility for Ella's care, I
capitulated to reality and placed her in the
Resources For Seniors Total Life Center (an
adult day center), two days a week. My
immediate sense of relief, and ability to totally
relax for the first time in several years, seems
proof of my need for and benefit from caregiver
respite. I believe Ella has perked up some, too,

since having periodic group interaction and stimulus from persons other than myself.

But I have unresolved issues. I need more than an occasional break from the daily tasks. I need support – emotional support – in this long-term grind. What's the answer?

Ken Wilber, in **Grace and Grit**, an autobiography on his wife's experience of breast cancer, and her subsequent death, puts the caregiver's dilemma graphically:

> "Nobody is interested in 'chronic'. What I mean is ... support people eventually begin to find their private problems are multiplying... They begin to feel completely alone and isolated. At this point, one of several things tends to happen. They walk out; they break down; they get into substance abuse; or they seek professional help.
>
> As I said, by far the best place to talk out your difficulties is in a support group for caregivers. When you listen to these groups, you find out that the main activity is basically griping about the loved ones. You know, 'Who does he think he is to order me around like that?' 'What makes her think she's so special, just because she's sick; I got problems of mine own, you know.' 'I feel like I've totally lost control of my life.' Those kinds of things nice people don't say in pulic, and certainly don't tell the loved one.
>
> The thing is, under all these dark feelings and anger and resentment is almost always a great deal of love, or else the support person would simply have walked out long ago. But this love can't really surface freely as long as

anger and resentment and bitterness clog the route..... There is a lot of hatred expressed in support groups, but only because there is so much love under it, starved love."

So there you have it: My situation, precisely. Could it be yours, also? Ella now has her group. And, I'm looking for MY support group too, to help me free up the love that I have for her.

Consider your need for respite assistance in caring for YOUR loved one. Look for the help of family; seek a support group in which you are able to free yourself for both loving and caring for that person you have committed to. Perhaps Resources For Seniors (or a similar helping agency) can assist you in finding respite, within or outside the home. Explore their resources for various caregiver groups.

Realize, as I have, that you cannot go it alone. This can be a truly freeing insight.

After writing this column, I took my own advice. The next week, I joined a caregiver's support group, sponsored and run by Resources for Seniors. The group meets every two weeks, and I have been able to ventilate my frustrations, see where others are coming from, and get a number of valuable tips on issues I was concerned about.

Breakout

A massive ice floe softens as the spring air warms the Arctic Ocean. Rumbling noises within the pack ice signal an impending annual event: the initial split across the seemingly solid ice mass. Within hours, the floe fractures into progressively smaller and smaller chunks, all the while melting and mixing with the ocean deeps. A cold, rigid, impenetrable physical presence is again returning to its elemental fluid nature: Water.

Another picture: A mass of logs, floating downstream, turns into one big jam when a single log turns crosswise at a point where the river narrows. In a dangerous maneuver, a lumberjack stands on the river of logs and pries the contrary beam away from its jammed position. With a jerky noise, the pack of logs resumes its journey downstream. The lumberjack, hopefully, scampers safely ashore.

These two metaphors touch upon a wonderful event involving my brother, two sisters and myself, back in April of 2000.

Over a span of fifty-plus years, Pearl, Jerry, Mary Ann and I had each married and moved apart, both geographically and interest-wise. At best, we had never been emotionally close; and time and circumstance had conspired to widen that gap considerably. Oh, we had annual family reunions for years, especially when the children were young, and our mother was still living. But, as the children left the nest, they attended family gatherings more and more sporadically. Reunions became less and less frequent. Then Mother died in 1994, and our last compelling reason to get together disappeared. The most recent reunion had been in 1996, after Jerry's wife, Mae, died, and he had remarried. "Now", I thought, "We may never come together again, as both Pearl and I have taken on caregiver roles for our respective spouses, and Jerry avoids all long trips, due to back problems."

Then, behold: A wondrous series of seemingly impossible events that turned into a breakout weekend!

Daughter Alice and her husband, Bill Hough, were celebrating their wedding anniversary, as usual, at Atlantic Beach. **But** this year they could only use three days of their timeshare. Alice says to me, " You haven't had any time off for a year, and you look tired. Would you like the condo for the other three days? I'll stay here with Mom while you're gone." As I eagerly answered, "Yes", she further suggested I might invite my sister, Mary Ann and husband, Carlton, for the trip. "And I might get them to pick up Pearl and bring her along, too", I quickly replied. This thing, in a matter of minutes, had snowballed into an almost-reunion, **if** Mary Ann and Pearl said, "Yes". Mary Ann and Carlton **did** say "Yes"! "And, we'll pick up Pearl, if she wants to come along." A phone call to Pearl: "Yes, I'll go. I need the time off from Brad (confined to a nursing home bed and wheelchair). Call Jerry and see if he can come." I'm almost breathless. I call Jerry: "Frances and I will be delighted to be with you and the others. I'll get a reservation nearby, and we can stop along the way, so I can rest my back." Wonder of wonders. It was really on!

We met at the condo, as planned. Jerry and Frances had a suite in the same facility. A breakout it was, indeed! For two days we refreshed our memories and emotional ties; experienced healing and reconciliation; reminisced – joked – laughed – even cried about our respective losses: Jerry's loss of Mae in 1996; Pearl's loss of close camaraderie with Brad, following heart attacks and strokes, and subsequent loss of speech and confinement to the nursing home; my similar loss of close connection with Ella, after years of oxygen deprivation and the 1997 stroke. In all of this, there seemed to be a most relaxed and unguarded atmosphere; and, at times, a kind of spontaneous joy that I hadn't experienced with them before.

When our "happening" was over, all four of us expressed a desire to renew our family relationship, this time as both blood kin and friends, who support each other through thick and thin! I **do** hope we can maintain this friendship and commitment in the future. I will do my part to see that we gather again.

Years 2001 and 2002 have seen us make that annual pilgrimage again, the last two times to a cousin's cottage at Nags Head, North Carolina.

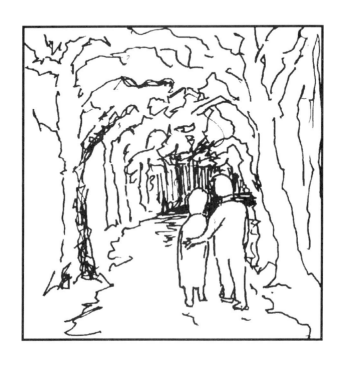

"Yea, though I walk through the
valley of the shadow of death, I will
fear no evil..."
Psalm 23:4
Bible, King James Version

On Caregiving: End Stage

Potholes and Pitfalls

May 11, 2000

Today was another milestone in Ella's journey along the road called sarcoidosis. She was accepted for Hospice of Wake services, to care for body and soul as she moves through the final miles of a long, treacherous and exhausting illness. I can no longer bear, alone, the increasing pressures of long-term caregiving. I am finally into the acceptance mode of my grieving for my love.

For eleven years, her lung air sacs gradually but insidiously were smothered by scar tissue, from an autoimmune process rare and little understood by the medical profession. Over the past five years, Ella's affliction has been more clearly manifested, with the gradual shutoff of blood oxygen – life's precious fuel, which stokes the body's furnace, powers muscles and other organs, and sustains the all-essential brain. Little wonder that she is now robbed of memory, and of most thinking ability. What remained of a sharp mind and keenly intuitive nature, after the stroke of '97 further compounded problems, was largely emotion – until last fall. Now, even this is fading, along with voluntary control of vital body functions. I weep as I see her dissolve before my eyes.

Which brings me to the issue of caring for the caregiver: In eleven years of advocating for and taking care of Ella, I've hit almost all of the possible potholes on that bumpy road; and every once in a while a sinkhole the size of my whole life has loomed ahead, and I've had to frantically steer my course in a different direction, to avoid disaster. One thing I've learned: Caregivers grieve, even as all of us grieve, at lost health, lost opportunities, lost relationships, and ultimately loss through death. I've visited those "stages" of grief – denial and isolation, anger, bargaining, depression, and acceptance – only to revisit each again and again, until the message comes through, loud and clear, and I am finally able to truly **accept** my wife's condition and imminent death. And as I watch the dying process, I still grieve.

When she was first diagnosed in January of 1989, I (and she) felt she had many years, before the sarcoid would incapacitate her. The right medication, prednisone, would keep the autoimmune process quiet; and she would continue at that 1989 level indefinitely. NOT SO! When her lung function rapidly deteriorated in 1995, and Ella went on oxygen, there was a lot of underlying anger, on the part of both of us. All along, I was bargaining with God, and the health professionals, for her to have as many healthy years as possible. As Ella lost physical and mental capacities, we both sank into despairing depression. No more quick fix. No more long-term plateau of the disease process. My weight ballooned; my emotional state sank; and my blood pressure and heart rate began to rise, ominously. Counseling and a weight-loss program put me back into physical balance, and moving toward acceptance of life-as-is, even as Ella continued to lose ground with the sarcoidosis and the residuals of the stroke(s).

But, the past six months have seen me revisit denial/anger/bargaining/depression many times. From day to day, my mood has swung wildly from deep despair, to detachment, to great optimism for my life, then again to despondency. Two days after making the decision to seek Hospice assistance – essentially agreeing to Ella's terminal condition in the near future – I developed a severe hives condition, body-wide. Two weeks later, the hives is finally subsiding, symbolic, I believe, of my final acceptance of her condition, and also of my acceptance of the needed help in these final days.

Oh yes. A rainbow in the sky, in the midst of the storm! I found a gem of a person to help Ella each morning with bathing, dressing, grooming, etc. Donna came into our lives just last Tuesday; and, already, I feel like a two-ton load has been lifted from my back!

Potholes galore, and pitfalls narrowly missed. But we both can see the rainbow, arched brilliantly across the road. And I am thankful for all those rough spots, which have taught me so much these last eleven years!

Surviving And Thriving

June 13, 2000

Another milestone occurred in Ella's life just two weeks ago. The pulmonologist recommended against her return to the Wellness Center exercise program. So, her final session there was last Wednesday, a "graduation" ceremony from the program, with a certificate of participation, a card full of well wishes from the class and staff; and a summary of almost five years of exercises: The number of classes attended, cumulative amount of weight lifted, cumulative miles walked. A monumental testimony, indeed, to a resolute lady's effort to overcome severe disability and remain active in all that life offers!

Now, my helpmate is more of a "shut-in" than ever before, although she still attends the Total Life Center in a wheelchair and is restricted to non-exercise activities there, too. Soon, that may also be denied her...and I become the "Help-Meet" for **all** her needs, in a closed-in world. How do I survive under such circumstances? Should I even think the word, "thrive"?

Luckily, I continue to have the counseling psychologist's weekly one-to-one support, to deal with the daily pressure-cooker atmosphere, and all the ups and downs. Then, too, I have the monthly long-term caregiver's group at Total Life Center, where more specific

27

long-term care issues are explored. These help me to survive.

But, life is more than just survival. Yes, as I move along on my emotional roller coaster and experience periods of turmoil, I **do** have to find a way to pay homage to a life so gallantly lived and now making its exit. I **do** honor her for all she has meant to me. In the same instant, I also have to find a way to maintain my own identity, in the midst of the present storm, as well as when Ella has finished her battle and passed on to her new life.

My Christian faith gives me compassion and a belief in Ella's and my continued life beyond this one. It may help me in the long term. But, what I need now is something to center me, give me emotional balance and calm, when our/my world is changing by the minute.

Which brings me to the "Tiger Woods" phenomenon of this past week: In the midst of the tempest of high-pressure pro golf, with all the possibilities of succumbing to self-doubts, moment-to-moment decision-making tensions, and media/crowd distraction, this 24 year-old son of a Thai-Buddhist mother and American father made history, by coolly playing his own golf game and refusing to self-destruct. Responding to the amazement of fellow professional golfers and the world-at-large, Tiger simply said, "I never felt unbeatable, but I had a...feeling of tranquility, of calmness. I was very much at ease with myself." He admits that he struggles to maintain that calm, but attributes much of his success to the

Buddhist practice of daily meditation and centering of his inner Self.

I believe that my own return to daily meditation, as well as prayer; a return to writing out my daily thoughts and feelings of self-recrimination, self-doubt and despair; and a daily release of all this negative, "bad" stuff to my God are a necessary step in my journey from mere survival to a life that thrives. The "Tiger Woods" story has impressed that on my psyche.

I once spoke of Ken Wilber's struggle with his wife's cancer and subsequent death. Speaking of his struggle to release his wife and move on with his own life, Wilber said,

> "...Treya's cancer is a constant reminder that death is a great letting go, but you needn't wait for actual physical death to profoundly let go of your own grasping and clinging to this moment, and this moment, and this."

I am resolved to do my letting go in these days and hours, so that I may not just survive an ordeal, but may both honor Ella's life **and** move on and thrive in my own future. I believe that is my lesson in this caregiving experience!

Personal and Up Front

July 19, 2000

In this series, I have tried to be personal and very specific about the caregiving challenges I've experienced with Ella's long-term disabilities and decline. Recognizing and dealing with the ups and downs of a disabled person's life makes for an interesting and exciting life for the caregiver – and an exhausting one, too!

Since retirement, much of my life has been devoted to giving Ella the needed care and support, while trying to reduce the jarring effect of daily crises, mood changes (both hers and mine), and the generally unpredictable nature of the illnesses, too. It's like being on a roller coaster, with its dips and sudden highs, but with that inevitable drop to the finish line. Half the anxiety is in not knowing when Ella is going to have a significant drop in physical function. In June, the pulmonologist says to her, "You've reached the point where the lung scarring is almost complete, and the medicine will no longer work efficiently. You will reach the point, in the not too distant future, when there will not be enough oxygen in the blood to keep the body going. How long that will be, I do not know." A real jolt to me, but I think she has taken it much more calmly than I.

Knowing that it will happen, but not knowing when, is the most difficult aspect of almost any illness. If it's a short, though intense, battle with the disease process, knowing there's an end point helps resolve the uncertainty, and therefore the constant tension. Long-term illness without a predictable pattern and a good sense of the time left makes for probably the most difficult situation.

I've previously described some of the personal "potholes" and "pitfalls" that I encountered, and how I've tried to deal with them. I also made a distinction between merely "surviving", and "thriving" in the midst of and in spite of the many adverse conditions. My next exploration into caregiving will raise other crucial issues most of us long-term caregivers will have to address: issues such as staying afloat, financially, for the long haul; keeping your dear one comfortable and with a sense that he/she is loved by you, the caregiver, to the end; involving the extended family in planning for and assisting in the loved one's long-term care, including preparing for death and all that implies.

This is only one person's journey. There are as many journeys as there are caregivers among us. May you share your caregiver journey with someone who needs it today!

An Afterthought: Come to think of it, I believe my wife became reconciled to her impending death eleven years ago, in early 1989, when the possible diagnoses ranged from tuberculosis, to cancer, to systemic pulmonary fibrosis and, finally, sarcoidosis of the lungs. Even then, when I asked her how she felt about the doctors' pronouncements, when cancer seemed the most likely diagnosis, Ella, with a kind of calm assurance, said she was ready to go, if that was to be her lot.

Of course, neither of us was prepared for eleven or more years of a chronic condition that wears down both the afflicted and the caregiver. I had watched my father deteriorate from multiple heart attacks, ulcers, and finally heart failure, after thirteen years. He passed in 1974, at age seventy-three. Ella's maternal grandmother suffered a massive stroke in 1929, at age sixty-nine, and was wheelchair-bound for twenty-five years. She was cared for by her husband, until the twenty-four hour a day, seven day a week load took him in 1944, at age eighty-six. The grandmother's care responsibility passed between Ella's parents and an aunt for the next ten years, until she died in 1954, ten days before our wedding.

Still, observing from the outside is not the same as living through the progressive disability. As person after person in our long-term care support group commented last Tuesday, "No one can realize the full impact of being incapacitated long-term, or of being the caregiver of such a person, until they are caught up in it themselves. You cannot 'tell it like it is', except to a person who has gone through it themselves." Wise words, indeed!

32

Points To Ponder

Bringing enduring meaning to this event called "The Caregiver's Journey", during a chronic illness that leads to death, is difficult. I've described the emotional roller coaster involved; daily stresses, wear and tear on body and soul; unceasing, moment-by-moment grieving. I've described the caregiver's monumental but necessary task of giving honor to the ill loved one and bringing about a separation between the two of them, thus releasing the helper to a new life. And, in the midst of this extended writing exercise, I continue to live the role I've tried to put flesh to.

Yet, I've neglected a couple of crucial issues that still have to be confronted, if the "Caregiver" event is to end on an upbeat or positive note. The first is financial survival. How to provide the loved one adequate care and still leave the caregiver with sufficient resources to live on, for the long haul?

I've done amazingly well this past year, considering my complete denial of the seriousness of our situation, until last October. I was like the proverbial mule that got a stick of wood up on the side of the head. But I finally got the message: Get your financial ducks in a row, or you're sunk! Finally, I got busy and had durable powers-of attorney for health and financial matters drawn up, for both Ella and myself. I also had a new will drawn up for myself, with a revocable trust added, so that if I passed first, Ella would be taken care of before my estate could be dispersed. I had living wills drawn up for each of us. Then, I segregated the funds and other assets, as allowed by law, after invoking the durable power-of-attorney for finances: I placed the house and auto in my name only; put our brokerage account in my name only; opened a credit union account in my name only, into which my annuity, Social Security, IRA distributions, and all broker distributions of interest and dividends now flow. Ella's retirement annuity and IRA distribution continue to go into our joint account, from which I can draw funds and issue checks for our mutual expenses. Hopefully, this strategy has given me maximum flexibility for income use, both before and after Ella's death.

But I was still in terror of the time I might have to place Ella in a facility. Much of our funds would be exhausted, should we have to qualify her for Medicaid, to pay for such care. Again, I resisted an obvious resource: Medicare's Hospice Program, dedicated to caring for Ella, and others like her, when the physician(s) can certify the likely terminal status of the patient within six months. Finally, I applied, and within two weeks Ella was certified as eligible for this cost-free (to us) program. As she spirals downward, week-by-week, I am, for the time being, relieved of excessive financial burden, although I still pay for meal preparation (evenings) and for bi-weekly maid service. Which brings me to the second crucial point in long-term care planning: Quality of life for the ill person, and a meaningful conclusion to that life, for the person, the spouse, the family, and all others concerned.

What Hospice means for us is hard to put into words: Each day, Ella has a home health aide help her from bed, bath and dress her (with back rub and lotion), and take her wheelchair to the table for breakfast. This is fully an hour eliminated from my former routine. Then, there are two visits a week by the nurse, to monitor Ella's medical status. All medications, certified as needed for the illness are provided free. Hospice-administered medications, for pain control are available. A social worker sees us every other week, also, for all sorts of needs. A chaplain visits, bi-weekly, for spiritual concerns. And a volunteer is available for several hours a week, for those times I must be out for shopping, etc. With this help, I can still have a life, apart from care-taking.

In connection with "quality of life", I have also placed a "Do Not Resuscitate" Order on our bedroom mirror, in the Total Life Center, and in the auto glove compartment. We'll have none of this 911 business! Ella wants to pass on while here at home! Finally, we are preparing now for her final memorial service: Ministers to officiate, poems to be read, songs to be sung, opportunities for personal memories, etc. Our sons and daughter are highly involved in these final months, and will be with us to the end.

Points To Ponder

We, as a couple, and as a family, have resolved to give meaning to Ella's life, so that it will not be a horror story to be forgotten, but an event of life-giving proportions. That is our deepest hope!

Postscript

October 17, 2000

No drama is complete without its denouement; no service of worship without a postlude; no letter to family or friend without its postscript, or afterthought. Likewise, the journey of a caregiver must reach a satisfactory resolution. Ella's death on September 14th, with its multifaceted aftermath, is teaching me that truth firsthand.

Despite our long-term anticipation and planning for the inevitable; the physical, emotional, and financial support of Hospice of Wake; and the blessed support of our children during those final months and weeks of Ella's illness, her death has still been a jarring rupture of life as it was for forty-six years: The daily, almost momentary, recall of last seeing her alive and then awakening to that moment of silent stillness, when I KNEW she was gone; the emotional crying jags of those first few days afterward; the sense of unreality, that I am now really alone.

The removal of Ella's body for cremation, in that first couple of dark hours; the calls next morning to family, friends, church; the final service plans reviewed with our Pastor; the completion of the written obituary, and placement with the News and Observer – these and many other activities filled that first day after. Friday saw the boys and their families arrive, as well as my siblings and their mates.

Postscript

Then there was the family and friends visitation in the Pullen Memorial Baptist Church Chapel, on Friday evening, for conversation and a visual presentation of the events and accomplishments of Ella's life, from childhood to a week before her death. Saturday's Memorial Celebration brought an upbeat end to a sorrowful three days. Songs, prayers, poetry, reflected memories of so many of her friends and relatives, and that finale of Ron Bell bagpiping Ella out of the Sanctuary to the tune of "Amazing Grace"! How can you beat that?

But the services are over, all the folks are gone home, and the house is empty, save this one. What to do with all the empty space – physical and emotional? What to do and feel, when awakening in the morning, reaching an arm across the bed – and nobody's there? What to do when a question forms in your mind, and the words die in your throat, as you realize there's no one to answer you? What to do with the dozens of visual reminders of a presence no longer physically with you?

It was a tough first week after Ella passed. But, luckily, the boys and their families were off, the following week, to an Edisto Island vacation, and I was invited, so I wouldn't continue to be alone. It was a time of physical and emotional recovery, with walks along the beach, family meals, and time to be alone and reflect on many things. And there was a time to write notes of appreciation to the many who had been there for us during "crunch time". Then it was back to the empty house...and the memories.

Postscript

I have begun to follow the advice of persons wiser than I, about adjustments needed so I can get on with life: Keep busy, but give yourself time to reflect, to grieve, to plan. Don't make big decisions for a while. Work gradually to change the living space into "your space". Think through carefully what to save of your departed loved one's belongings; cherish what is left.

Let the memories return, as they will. Laugh at those times that were so amusing; cry at the sorrows you shared; rise up in joy at those indescribable times of happiness and Spirit that wed you together as One!

Of course, you will work to create a lifestyle for one: Exercise and eat well, to stay healthy. Get out of the house daily, and meet and enjoy other people. Find, or continue activities that give you joy, and a sense of purpose. I could go on endlessly. But you get the picture: After death, there is life – Life in the Spirit for your Beloved – Life in the dual role of flesh and spirit, for yourself. Count yourself blessed to have known her/him. Cherish the memories. But, then make the break and find a new life for yourself. Life goes on!

A Memorial
to Ella

Together

From diverse sources, yet from one,
Wrought in Love o'er eons, once again we meet.

Two rivers flowing down separate beds.
We cascade, tumble, or amicably gurgle our way
along.
'Til two, in noisy delight now mingle,
ne'er again to completely part.

In past we fed on Life's Repast:
Still, once again we meet to share
Another Great Feast, Yours and Mine,
Divinely giv'n;
A Banquet, great gifts, pour out before our eyes.

And yet that greatest banquet
from God's Heart doth pour
Through Us, the simple Trinity of Life —
Companions, Friends, and Lovers always.

We come from diverse places, yet from One,
As streams from separate sources.
We blend lives, memories, thoughts, emotions,
to become a new mix of God's Living Bread.

Now blended, we move into Our Future.
We are as One Forever,
TOGETHER

Composed by Robert Jeter, in celebration of the
union of Deanna and Dan, August 28, 1999.
Read at the Celebration of the Life of Ella Hutchins
Jeter, September 16, 2000

To A Lovely Lady And Enduring Partner

September 15, 2000

Ella Hutchins Jeter. How does one put into a few words forty-six years of experiences with this extraordinary woman, the Love of my life? Impossible! Yet, try I must!

My first memory was of a broad smile from a winsome brunette, with a most fetching and beautiful face, as she handed out sandwiches and punch, across the counter of the Recreation Hall kitchen. The time was the fall of 1952; the place, Tabernacle Baptist Church, Raleigh, North Carolina. Our first date? It was around Easter, the following spring. After that, it was every Friday or Saturday evening, either for a movie at Five Points, or a dinner at a local restaurant. But, more often than not, it was just an evening in her living room, with Ella's parents conveniently elsewhere in the house. Within weeks, it was serious stuff!

Then it was long-distance dating, with two hundred and eighty mile Friday evening trips from Aiken, South Carolina, where I worked at an atomic energy facility, to Raleigh. Sunday evenings saw me headed back to Aiken.

We were married on a January evening in 1954, just after a major snowstorm. Many out of town guests never made it, including my Dad and sister Pearl. Ella's first major disappointment: There were only sixty plus

43

people at the service. I was standing there, shaking in my boots. Ella was calmly counting the "crowd". She had planned for up to 175 people. But life must go on! So we had a wedding, a reception at the Woman's Club, and then headed out for the rest of our lives.

Like most courting young ladies, my bride envisioned her Prince Charming. Instead, she got her frog - ME, warts and all. Still, she has made the best of bad times; has followed this vagabond from place to place, as I quickly burned up one vocation after another. As I would start another educational program, she would grit her teeth and then work with me to keep the family together: She worked while I went to seminary. We both took temporary jobs as I toughed out a Master's program in Rehabilitation Counseling in Richmond, Virginia. Then, when we were barely making ends meet in my DC vocational rehabilitation counseling job, and we had the chance to again own a home, Ella returned to the work force, as a secretary at Washington, D.C.'s Saint Elizabeth Hospital. Fifteen years later she would retire, as an Administrative Assistant, from her job in the Hospital Superintendent's office.

Ella retired in November of 1988. In early January, 1989, she was diagnosed as having sarcoidosis, an inflammation that was scarring her lungs, both restricting her breathing capacity and the effectiveness of oxygen-carbon dioxide exchange. Prognosis? Several good years, with the sarcoidosis held in check by medication. As the medication repeatedly lost its effectiveness, the lung alveolae would

44

continue to scar, Ella would become increasingly short of breath and eventually require an external source of oxygen. She had maybe ten to fifteen years of life left. Ella's reaction? "I know I have to die sometime. Let's live it while we have it!"

Six good years followed, of marrying off two sons, traveling, and watching and loving grandchildren arrive and begin their own journeys. Following our 1993 return to Raleigh, Ella went on oxygen in 1995. She also entered a pulmonary exercise class at Rex Wellness Center in October of 1995 and, for four and a half years, benefited immensely from it. She still enjoyed life, including church activities and visiting our families. In 1997, Ella's health further declined, with a mild stroke, which effectively shut her off from beloved activities of knitting, crocheting, and ceramic work.

Still, to the end, she persevered. She did for herself, until she could do it no more: When, in June, she could no longer attend Wellness Exercise Class, on doctor's advice Ella still attended the Total Life Center twice a week, as she had since November of 1999. When she became unable to stand and walk, two weeks ago, my Love was confined to the bed. Still, she refused to go quietly. For most of the last two weeks, Ella slept sitting on the side of the bed, resting with her head on a bedside tray table, with a pillow on it. To the end, she fought inactivity.

Yet, with all her infirmities, Ella Hutchins Jeter was one tough cookie! She was resolute,

45

in the face of adversity. Example: Over ten years, she was pregnant six times, spontaneously miscarrying three times. But, she has reared three lively and loving children, now sitting here, with spouses and their own children, to attest to her love of life. She was devoted to providing a strong parental model for each child.

Ella had a sharp wit, even to the end, to which Hospice folk can attest. To illustrate: Just last Wednesday, the day of her death, although seemingly unconscious when volunteer Betty Ann Corby entered, she suddenly opened her eyes; said matter-of-factly, "Oh, you're here"; smiled; then lapsed back into a sleep or unconscious state. How about THAT?

Another enduring characteristic was her giving. She gave, sometimes to a fault, when her own health was jeopardized. She gave to others in listening. She was a good listener. Oh, the many hours she spent in listening to friends, and holding them up in times of crisis! Ella was essentially a follower, not a leader. But as private as she was, she did not hesitate to voice strongly held convictions when asked for an opinion – much like her father, whom she adored and often turned to for advice.

Ella gave of her many crafted works, gifts to family, friends and neighbors, without reserve. A knitted sacque for a friend's or neighbor's newborn; a crocheted afghan to friends, old and young; crocheted Christmas stockings and snowflake ornaments for the tree. She cooked all kinds of nourishing meals and goodies, and shared them whenever she felt the person or family in need. She spent many hours at school functions, in the early years of our children's lives. She gave to me in ways that I could never repay... So much giving.

With all this serious stuff, one would think my frau didn't have time to enjoy life. Wrong! She enjoyed sitting with me, in the summer moonlight. She loved to sit at an open doorway and watch it rain and the lightning crackle, and listen to the thunder roll. We shared barefoot walks along the beach, searching for shells and other treasures of the sea. She loved hot chocolate and marshmallows, while watching it snow furiously on a cold winter day. She loved cooking solid, nourishing meals and delicious cakes, cookies, pies, etc, for a hungry and appreciative family.

Ella loved the personal moments between us: Watching a red evening fireball descend on the western horizon; the moonlight strolls; walking in the snow; our many "walkathons', in which she consistently left **me** gasping for air! Then, there were the mutual late evening backrubs for easing the aches of the day. And, yes, we loved the occasional weekend hot showers we shared, long before the ad men usurped this essentially spiritual but sensual image for their TV commercials!

A few other little tidbits: Ella was a yard sale and flea market nut. No trip was complete for her until we had made at least one, preferably more stops, where she might pick up a plate, a book, anything that suited her fancy. Although she bordered on dyslexia, my wife always had a book by the chair, which she would pick up when she was tired of knitting or crocheting. She collected plates, usually one of a kind. She collected bells, several dozen over the years. She collected owls and mushrooms, for her friend, Martha. She painted by the numbers. And, she collected teddy bears. There must be fifty or more little cuddle bears in the house by now!

So much more to share! And for every memory uncovered, a dozen more float to the surface.

Thus, I must somehow close this meandering walk down memory lane, but not without one final moving event. On Wednesday evening, around 11:00 PM, I last saw her living physical form, still panting somewhat for breath, despite the medication to ease this condition.

Just past 1:00 A.M., I awakened to a mysterious stillness. I looked at my Beloved. Completely still of body; no movement of face; no twitching of any muscle. I rose from the bed, came to her side of the bed, and facing the now still form, touched the face, searched for a pulse. Nothing. She was gone. Still, I was strangely quiet – sad, but not despairing. I had left the light on when I went into an exhausted sleep.

Now, I began to feel a lightness of heart, even as the light in the room took on a kind of glow. Now I KNEW! I looked at the lifeless body and said, out loud, "You're not in that body!" Then I looked up into that shimmering light that seemed to glow, even in the midst of the shadows. My next comment surprised me to the core. "You're up there, looking at me, and laughing at me."

My eyes turned further right and fixed on my long-deceased mother's watercolor of a majestic tern, wings spread into an invisible air, and just hovering ... just hovering. And a peace settled over my being. She is there, ALIVE, and one day, not too long from now, I'll be there, too!

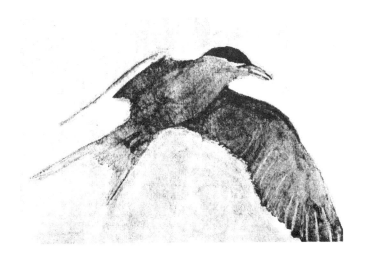

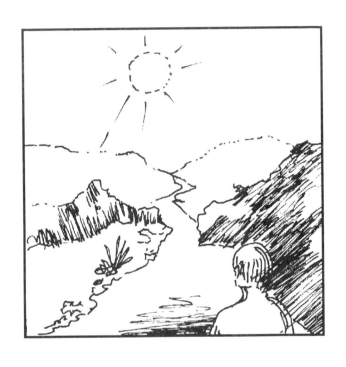

"Surely goodness and mercy will
follow me
all the days of my life..."
Psalm 23:6
Bible, King James Version

On Aftercare: Grief and Recovery

The Beat Goes On

November 17, 2000

I intended to close the caregiver series with last month's Postscript. But, still, the memories flow, and the words pour forth, out of my heart, from my mind and onto the paper. So, I will probably have more to say on caregiving over time, as new issues come to the foreground: Things such as how to make constructive personal adjustments, both immediately and for the long term. How to cope with one's loss and grief at meaningful times such as anniversaries and holidays. How to find personal meaning in life after the death of one whose life has been intertwined with ours, so deeply and for so long. So I presently plan to take up these vital concerns, probably in the order above stated.

My first concern is about how one can best get through the immediate impact of losing one's Significant Other. Thinking through the events of these tension-packed past six months, several images immediately come to mind: Words like Decompression, Aftershock, Boobytrap, Regrets, Remorse, Guilt, etc. The point of bringing up such ideas is to stress that such mental and emotion stirrings are normal and necessary to adequately and constructively grieve a major loss, like that of a spouse. Let me give a personal face to a few of these images.

Decompression: It is often difficult for me

to imagine the sense of lightness and release of pressure I felt, upon the death of this person I had cared for over many years. It seemed hard to accept that sensation as right and normal. So I, as caregiver, had some intense feelings of *Guilt:* Was it right for me to feel so relieved that the battle was over? Was I being uncaring, feeling that way? Again, at one point, I felt *Remorseful:* Did I do enough to care for my wife during her illness, to show my love and devotion to her? Then, there was the *Regret:* the heartrending pain, upon the realization I would have no further opportunity to redress my perceived lack of care for Ella. These are issues of the Heart and Soul that have no easy answer, and are easy to trip over. These become emotional *Boobytraps*, that can wound us, painfully and permanently, if not recognized as such and carefully avoided.

Then I began to feel that I was over the hump, that I was now successfully putting some emotional distance between myself and my departed wife, only to have images and feelings spontaneously well up, as an overwhelming tide. The *Boobytrap* – again. It keeps happening, so often and at such unpredictable times! And, then comes *Aftershock*. Some of my friends describe how, even many months and years later, these grief reactions again return, to at least temporarily prostrate them. I had this experience, two months after Ella's death, on her birthday, November 7th. She would have been seventy-five that day. I've been told to expect more of the same, come Thanksgiving, Christmas, and especially our forty-seventh wedding anniversary, January 23rd.

So, I've experienced these things. I've been counseled by friends to expect a rough year, or more. And I've been assured, by persons who have been through my kind of experience: *I will survive.* A most comforting thought!

In the meantime, I'm filling the vacuum with things I did before Ella's passing: I'm attending Hospice of Wake's seven week Caregiver's Grief Support Group, a priority for awhile. I'm bowling, twice weekly. I'm going to my exercise program M-W-F, each week. I'm writing for Senior Source, and resuming work on a novel. I'll be clowning at a few events, over the next few months, maybe. And, I'm helping prepare Wednesday Night Suppers at my church; eating and visiting with my friends, there; and resuming my place in the Choir Loft on Sundays. Holidays will be spent with the family. A full schedule, and yet I haven't taken on any new projects, just yet.

But give me time to adjust to the new lifestyle, and renew my physical vitality! There are some new projects in the air, some coming attractions. Ella's New Life issues in. My Life continues, here. The Beat Goes On!

Grief And Advent

December 15, 2000

On December 15th, I walk into an empty house. The only stimuli are the low roar of the air-handler and a sensation of warm air blowing across the floor. I immediately think, "Ella's not here, to share my pleasure in having a good day at bowling." Once again, a real downer! The answering machine light is blinking. A new message, which I immediately check: "This is Christena Schafale, Senior Source Editor. I know it's a couple of days early, but I'll be leaving for Christmas vacation next Friday and need your Pot Pourri article in by Monday, so I can have it to the printer before I leave."

Hmm.... I've been putting it off, as usual, claiming all sorts of reasons (excuses). I've been too busy, blah, blah, blah. Then, I recognize a real resistance to writing anything for a drab winter month, like February, when my mood is so down. I think to myself, "Writing for others, from this low energy level and depressed mood, will be about as much fun as having a tooth pulled. All I'll accomplish will be to make them depressed, too. I've been working real hard on owning my residual feelings for the past six weeks, through the Hospice Grief Support Group. These feelings are still fresh and raw. I just don't know what I should do about the column."

As often happens when I need direction on

an issue, I head for the great outdoors. I pull on my sweater, windbreaker and stocking cap. With umbrella under an arm, I head out for a walk in the 40-degree night air, under cold-looking cloud-covered skies. I expect this trip to be a chore, the damp and inky night to reflect back my feelings of loss and aloneness. What a surprise! A kind of warmness immediately creeps over me, as I stretch out my limbs down the first block of my mile and a third trek. It's really invigorating! And, it takes away, at least temporarily, that edgy tension with which I've become so familiar these past three months since Ella's death.

Another revelation, as I walk my walk: Christmas is just around the corner, and I've only half-heartedly decorated the living room, with a creche, red candles, and Ella's ceramic Christmas tree, all lighted up. The plastic wreath is on the outside of the storm door. The one real enthusiasm I've had in this process is when I put Ella's crocheted and starched Angel on top of that lighted ceramic tree. A first time for the Angel, since coming to Cary! Now, curiously, during my walk I begin to take notice of many homes that are all lit up, in various themes and patterns. In my head, I'm prepared to do my Ebenezer Scrooge "Bah Humbug", about all the gaudiness of the lighted neighborhood.

Despite all my premeditated skepticism at the commercialism and crassness of Christmas, the words "Advent" and "Immanuel" slip into my consciousness. Then the idea that I have already had and continue to have my personal "Advent" presses on me. I hark back to Ella's desperate days of illness, just before her death, and see and hear all the many "Angels of Mercy", from Rex Wellness Center, Total Life Center, Hospice of Wake, Pullen Memorial Baptist Church, who ministered to her. I remember the love and devotion that Alice, Lee and Al showered on their mother over the years, and their special attention to her needs as the end neared. I find priceless Ella's brother, Ed Hutchins, and his wife, Nell, whose prayers and deeds of love have been spread over our lives for many years. We have been prayed for and assisted by many others of Ella's family, as well as my own kin. I remember our personal helper, Donna Sousa, who fed us with food **and** conversation for the last, crucial four months, and who still assists me with meals a couple of times a week. These, and so many other unacknowledged "Angels" were and are our "Advent", the coming of the Christ into our lives. I still experience a personal "Advent" or "God with Us", as so many of these good folk continue their ministry to the children and me.

Ending this walk, I remember these many evidences of "God with Us", with a joy and enthusiasm not present when I started out. As I re-enter the house, I remove my wraps and prepare some hot spiced apple cider. Then, I turn on the computer and begin to write about our/my "Advent" and "Immanuel", God-with-Us, just ten days before the official celebration. Joy to the World!

What Are You Waiting For?

January 16, 2001

That's exactly what I've been asking myself for the past several weeks, now that I've survived the Holidays! Of course, I'm referring to my efforts to move on with my life since Ella's death. It's not that easy though. I will think I've worked through most of the grief, cried my eyes dry, and then someone tells of a personal loss, or a poignant story is aired on radio or TV, and it starts all over again.

Gratefully, the depression is lifting, I weep less often, and I begin to see more and more humor in life situations. The mountains of loss and loneliness seem much lower these days. Lately, I've answered the inquiries of folks, "How are you doing?" with "I'm almost over the hump." That's it! That mountain is becoming more like a molehill. I'm almost over the hump. Another BIG hill is just ahead – our forty-seventh anniversary, on January 23d. But, with the help of family and friends, I should get over that hump, too.

So, what else am I waiting for right now? One thing I've been putting off is writing this Pot Pourri, which is in the process of resolution, even now as I write these words. OK. What other things still await my decision and action?

Back in early October, I had made

application for a part-time job as a Center Aide at the new Cary Senior Center. At that time, there was no way I would have been able to deal with the pressures of the job. However, Center Director Jody Lindsey, in her wisdom and compassion, let me cool my heels for several months. Then, she interviewed me this week. Now, I feel much stronger and focused for adequately performing the job I was offered. I should begin training and active duty at the Senior Center within a week or two.

Other challenges? This week, it's back to bowling and T'ai Chi. Then there's the new Lite Aerobics Class, offered M-W-F at Cary Senior Center, as well as an every other Thursday Reader's Theatre Session there, also.

Within another month or so, I may also be ready to get back into clown mode. I've been back in church choir since November. You say to me, "Whoa there! How are you going to keep up with all this activity?"

Well, remember that story I told awhile back, about me and that calendar battling it out for priority time? A year ago, it was all I could do to keep Ella's Wellness Center, Total Life Center, and medical treatment appointments coordinated, and get her from place to place on time, week in and week out. Add to that seeing to oxygen equipment and supplies, and weekly church services, and I had precious little time and energy to "do my thing". Still, I was able to get in the exercise, T'ai Chi and bowling. I had dropped choir, back in the summer of 1997.

What Are You Waiting For?

This time around, the calendar has been full of blanks, which I've filled in with personal priority items first – exercise, recreation, music, drama, clowning and Carolina Health and Humor Association events. The part-time job fits into the remaining free weekday and evening hours very nicely. And I have committed to try reading to a class of kindergarten students, for an hour once a month, at Wiley Magnet School, in Raleigh. This is something I've put aside for a long time. Now, it's time I give back to the children.

So, what am I waiting for? Certainly not for someone to pull me out of the house, so I don't mope around forever! There are kids to be taught and inspired, the ill to be served a little humor in their diet, the lonely to be cheered. And, I have lessons of my own to learn from all this, too. Things are about to start a-popping again! Thank God for good things to do!

On
Reconnection

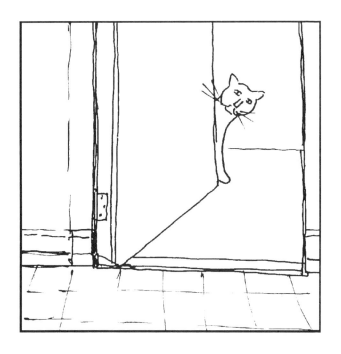

You're The Cat's Meow!

March 29, 2001

It was in late November, a couple of months after Ella's death. I had never seen this cat before, but there she was: An ash gray tabby cat, with emerald green eyes, and the most inquisitive, appealing stare that I had ever seen! Whose little feline she was, I had no idea, but she obviously belonged to someone in the nearby neighborhood. She was too sleek, and looked too well fed not to.

I've never been very close to pets, especially cats, but now I had this particular cat almost every day, in my driveway or on the sidewalk, where I couldn't help either passively walking around her or, more actively, shooing her onto the grass. She would even run after me, onto the deck, and try to follow me into the house, as if she was saying, "This is my house, too. Let me in!" It happened, not once or twice, but two or three times a week, from late November through February.

Because I didn't want to encourage this newcomer to come into my now much emptier world, I never put a hand on "Kitty". She might **really** take up with me, make me her owner and companion, and I wasn't ready for that. Still, "Kitty" appealed to me by various subterfuges. Sometimes it was a coy kind of approach, in the way she would cock her head to one side and give me a questioning stare, much as if to say, "Don't you like me? Please

63

pay attention to me!" Again, it would often be a much bolder approach, like coming to the open front door and intently looking inside the glass storm door. If I didn't pay any attention to her, that cat would then look straight at me, "Meow", then scratch energetically on the clear glass.

There were some days when I would head out the front door, only to find this "Kitty" on the deck, barring my exit. If I shoved against her, she would back off a few feet and roll over on her back, literally asking me to bend down and rub the fur on her belly. I never did. But, interestingly, I began to strike up a conversation with "Kitty", on a regular basis, like I might be talking to Ella or someone else. "What are you doing here, this time? You still think you can coax me into petting you and letting you into the house. You sure act like you own this place. I do believe you even think you own **me!**" All this while I headed for the car and the cat loped behind me and tried to crawl into the vehicle. It got so that she would head out ahead of me and jump on the hood of the car, even before I could get there, unlock the door and get in. If I happened to open the car window for a little air, my self-appointed furry companion would try to crawl into the auto through that open window space. And on many occasions, when I came back home and turned off the engine, "Kitty" would jump up on the hood and take advantage of the warmth – sort of like coming in out of the cold and curling up next to a hot air duct! I got so I was quite curious what this feline would do next.

By March, I had again begun to fill my life

with both meaningful people and activities. Then, all of a sudden, "Kitty" stopped her daily drop-ins. I might see her from afar, but that was the extent of it. I put the question to her, and to myself: "Where have you been? Why haven't you been around?" And I realized I missed her, very much! But not as much as I would have, had she not insisted on joining me, as "family", in those early days of bereavement. It was then that I realized how this cat had come into the life of a very lonely man, and given me some much needed companionship at just the time I needed someone, something to be there.

I sincerely believe that God directed "Kitty" to my doorstep, when I needed her most. A kind of insistent voice that said, "There's still Life out here, even if you don't think so. Give Life a chance to come back into your heart."

Thank you very much, Kitty. You're the "cat's meow"!

A Healing Touch

May 13, 2001

I said, in my last column or two, that I was
about finished with "The Caregiver's Journey"
series. And then "You're the Cat's Meow"
popped right up in the front of my conscious
focus. Now, **another** of those moments! But,
this one took some percolation before the whole
story brewed to a nice, pleasant flavor!

First, a brief explanation: In beginning Pot
Pourri, some four and a half years ago, one of
the "rules" impressed on me was that I should
not impose my personal religious perspective
and feelings on my readers. By and large, I
have attempted to keep my views religiously
neutral, even in "The Caregiver's Journey".
Still, aspects of The Journey continue to
impose themselves on **me.** Let me describe the
particulars.

Usually, an idea pops into my head, and
with it an apt title. But, this time, I have been
waiting...and waiting...and waiting. No ready
topic came to mind for the July issue. "What is
going on here?" I asked myself. Questions
arose, like "Is the well running dry? Is my
other writing project, a major work, draining
me of energy and inspiration for the Senior
Citizen's point-of-view at this particular time
and place in my life? What's blocking me from
seeing, feeling, experiencing something
valuable to impart to my monthly audience?"

A Healing Touch

I was most frustrated yesterday, right up to bedtime, so I took special care to ask my God and my personal Muse or Genius to speak to me in my sleep. Please give me **something** to share with the reader this month! It took me a while to drift off, but finally I entered a deep sleep. Then my slumber became light and fitful, and a series of dreams began – impressions of an aloneness, a desire for my love to again be by my side.

I must admit that previous conscious pleas had not been much help in restoring to me a sense of Ella's conscious presence. The eight months since her death had led to a gradual distancing of my heart's feelings, and my mind's imagination from her physical reality. She was physically dead, and although real in my faith's eye, Ella had become only a dim whisper in my Mind and Soul.

Then, this experience! The loneliness, the aloneness became an overpowering feeling, even in the dream state. I struggled to awaken. And then...then, a whole new feeling arose, that she was there. As the mist of dream-state slowly dissolved, I heard three low, distinct words calling out to me: "Bob...Bob...Bob...." Then the dream was gone and I was awake, with my left arm draped across the right side of the bed where once she had slept, and where we had discussed, argued and loved one another.

No physical Ella. But I swear I could sense her presence once again, even down to "seeing" her physical form and smelling the delicate scent of her cologne, her distinctive bodily aroma. "She is here again!" I exclaimed. Then I remembered this just-passed Mother's Day, when I picked a lovely, pinkish white peony from our front yard, pinned it to my gray silk jacket, and headed for the morning worship service. Just as I had been sad and "down in the dumps" on Mother's Day of 1997, when Ella had suffered that first serious stroke, the prelude to the long "Caregiver's Journey", this later day I went forth bright and all buoyed up.

And, suddenly, I had a compelling urge to depart the bed and head for the computer and tell my story. And here I am, at 8:00 AM, on the 13th day of May, 2001, words exploding upon the computer screen and soon to be on the printed page for your eyes, too. The message? Ella and I still walk down that road of life, toward the sunset of my own earthly existence. And, I, too, shall walk through that thin veil we call "Death", just like it's a foggy mist.

And you will see me no more. But, I'll be on the other side, walking hand in hand with my Ella, and we will laugh...and cry...and love... and commune with each other once more. Of that I am once more assured.

Peace to All.

Surviving The Fire

August 21, 2001

(In reviewing the original version of this article for inclusion in this book, I have become aware of a continuing anger at the loss of Ella, a heat still smoldering beneath the surface of my veneer of coolness. It's much like the heat radiating from a just-ejected flow of lava. So, I am now reworking this account, that I may give greater emphasis to my increased awareness of the inner dynamics of grief. Here are my revised, most up-to-date thoughts and feelings on the issue. -- July 22, 2002)

In the most literal sense, this story has been on the back burner ever since my wife's death. At its deepest level, this has to do with a ravishing fire.

Fire: the great destroyer and consummate purifier. In Greek mythology, Prometheus was punished for stealing fire from the Gods, and Icarus was destroyed when he heedlessly came too close to the sun. Biblically speaking, the Refiner's Fire burns away the worthless dross of one's life and lets the luster of the remaining gold shine through. Poetically, A. S. Coleman pictures the black man (and by analogy, his soul) as like tall trees that remain standing after a fierce forest fire. I also have had my encounter with fire.

First of all, out of my family lore arises the

story of my grandmother's tenant farmhouse
twice burned to the ground, once in the dead
of winter. It was during Mother's early
childhood, and made such an enduring
impression on her that she told the story
endlessly to her own offspring.

All this is further etched upon my
consciousness by a personal experience from
my 1940's high school days. I was a member of
the student chapter of Future Farmers of
America. One day, we were trying to put out a
fire in a southeastern Virginia woodland.
Although it was only a small ground fire, I can
remember vividly my growing apprehension,
almost to the point of panic, as the flames
seemed to be racing beyond the control of our
picks, shovels, rakes and portable water
spraying equipment. In more recent years, I've
watched the great western fires on TV, with
great empathy for the fearsome task that so
many firefighters face, as they suppress and
subdue the raging flames coursing through
treetops and up narrow canyons. What heart-
stoppers are these monster fires, consuming
all in their paths!

Yet there are emotional fires of equal
ferocity racing through the being of each
person who ministers to a dying spouse,
relative or friend; watches that loved one pass
on; and then tries to comprehend, with heart,
mind and soul, the immensity and
permanence of that loss. As I approach the
first anniversary of Ella's death, both body and
mind have been reminding me of that loss. I
have found myself having to consciously
remember her face and voice, her touch, even

her physical smell. I have had that internal panic, that I might lose all that emotional and physical memory.

Along with the immediate, dynamic, visceral, emotional relationship that we enjoyed, I have missed the shared conversations, even our periodic times of confrontation. Those were the times when we expanded our spirits, individually and as a couple. I have felt bad about our many missed opportunities for mutually exploring our Spirits and bringing them closer to the one Spirit we envisioned at the time of our marriage. So, with Ella's passing, there have been great firestorms raging through **my** Spirit – storms of despondency, of despair; fires of guilt feelings over lost chances for reconciliation and growth. So many great fires of the Soul!

Yet my Spirit still lives, burned and scorched on the surface but still vital and growing within. I liken it to the cataclysmic eruption of Mount St. Helens, back in the '80s: a third of the mountain blown away and the flora of the entire area burnt to seeming oblivion, for twenty to thirty miles in every direction. The "experts" said it would be many years before life returned to the mountain. Now, only a decade or two later, life flourishes there again with renewed vigor and splendor.

Many folks will be saying that we widows and widowers will never recover our vigor or our splendor. But remember: we are like those tall trees that still stand after the raging fires have died away. From what I've experienced in

the last year, I'd say those folks don't know
what they're talking about.   They have to go
through the fire, like we have. Then and only
then will they have the right or authority to say
anything!

When Does Closure Come?

September 21, 2001

"Closure": The magic word, the buzz-word of the 1980's and the 1990's. A word that many think implies an end to whatever shackles us to the past; more specifically, a complete emotional resolution that frees one from anger, guilt, or anything else that imprisons him or her in a negative situation. "Closure" implies leaving the past behind and moving on freely into the rest of one's life.

I thought I was close to closure. I had grieved my loss of Ella and was on the way toward wholeness, health, and a thoroughly positive move into the future. And then a modern version of the four apocalyptic horsemen – War, Fear, Famine and Death – intruded on the reality of myself and all other Americans. They came in the form of four aircraft converted by kamikaze hijackers into lethal bombs that destroyed the New York World Trade Towers and severely damaged the Pentagon in Washington, DC – and with that came the death of the hijackers and passengers on all four planes. Most heinously, these planes and their misguided, demented and hate-filled captors took with them the lives of countless innocent persons. As I write these words, the missing and dead count for the World Trade Towers alone is initially estimated at more than six thousand. Many more are injured.

Oh, the irony of it! I rolled into Kitty Hawk, NC at 12:15 PM, Tuesday, September 11th, to give the remains of Ella's cremated body to the Atlantic Ocean, on the first anniversary of her death. Since the auto radio had been turned off, that I might have silence for meditation, the horrible revelation still awaited me. Alighting from the car, I was immediately greeted by the disaster news, via an emotionally distraught sister, Pearl. My anticipated emotional closure, through this symbolic personal ritual of releasing my beloved's ashes to the great ocean of God's love was instantly diluted, tainted by a great sorrow, shared by so many. But I determined to do that task which I had come to complete at this natural sanctuary.

So, I waited for the dawning of the 12th, then arose, drove down close to Duck Road Beach and exited the car, to the mighty roar of crashing waves. I removed from the back seat of the auto a clear plastic bag, heavy with white to dark gray ashes. The walk over the dunes and down to the white ocean sands was a mere hundred yards or so, into a blazing sun, rising in all its glory on a clear eastern horizon. The landscape, consonant with my own emotional turmoil, was filled with angry, white-capped waves, four to five feet high, and a twenty mile per hour wind that rippled across the sea oats. Dry sand blew against my body and face. In solemn reflection, I kicked off my sandals and slowly descended to water's edge and let the dying surge lap up over my feet. Cautiously, I descended until feet were

submerged to the ankles. The cool and salty
Atlantic, like unto the great ocean of God's
Love, calmed my thinking and feelings.
Looking at the ashes and saying a prayer, I
slowly opened the bag, turned its open end
downward and gently sifted the gray matter
into the surging and ebbing water. As I
watched the fine particles sink into the water
and disperse with each ebbing wave, I looked
up into the sun-drenched sky and wished my
Ella Godspeed, into the Great Mystery of the
life beyond. After some five minutes, I backed
onto the dry sand of the upper beach, still in
meditation. Then I returned to the car.

Later that morning, I went back to Duck
Road Beach, walked the sands for another
half-hour and took pictures of the violent
ocean and the sunlight shimmering across its
surface. While I was turned toward the sea, at
some point I became aware of a presence.
Looking behind me, I came face to face with a
gray-white seagull, standing no more than
fifteen feet away. It stared at me in all its
majesty. And I thought of my feeling of Ella's
presence with me the night of her death, when
I looked upon the painting of the soaring tern,
next to my bed. As I left the beach this time, a
feeling of peace settled over mind and body,
over my very being. For the first time, I felt
some genuine closure. That peacefulness
remains to this moment.

Closure is never complete, picture-perfect.
I have learned that a measure of personal
closure allows me to go on. But the memories
remain, the ache comes back periodically, the
loss is never completely forgotten. Our great

national tragedy also bears on me, moment to
moment, and I have to deal with its grief and
pain, just as I did during those World War II
years...and the many wars and tragedies since.
Just as I now remember...and grieve...and
ache with Ella's passing. But, in all the
hurting, all the pain, there arises another
enduring emotion: Gratitude, for **all** of Life's
experiences! Out of the sorrows have come the
emotions with which to feel Love and Joy.
Thanks Be to God!

On Life Anew

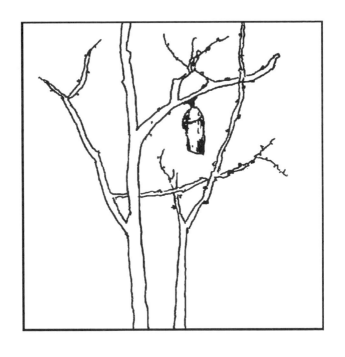

Testing The Waters

January 20, 2002

You walk up to an icy-looking pond or pool of water, ready to take the plunge, but dreading that initial, frosty shock. Someone already immersed and obviously enjoying the swim, says, "Come on in, the water's fine. It's warmer here than in that cold air out there." But you're not so sure they're right. You've never been one to jump into anything without first testing it. So you creep up to water's edge and slowly, ever so s-l-o-w-l-y, stick your big toe into the fluid. Reflexively, you yank it back, teeth chattering. Your companion in the water says, "Come on! Come on in! It's better to just jump right in. It gets warmer, once you're wet." Finally, shivering all over and your heart racing, you hold your breath and make the leap. Bobbing up to the surface, after the initial shock subsides, you begin to stir around, first doing a gentle dog paddle, then shifting into the slow rhythm of the Australian crawl. Finally, you flip over, face up, and leisurely begin the backstroke.

What's this all about? It's a parable on the predicament of someone who needs a little reassurance in returning to the waters of single life. Which is where I am presently, now eighteen months into the state of widowhood.

The initial plunge was when I finally took Ella's ashes to the waters of Southern Shores, NC, and emotionally released both her body and spirit to the keeping of our God. Since then, the waters of my new life have been warming up, day by day.

First off came several defining decisions: I sold the Craftmatic bed we had shared for seventeen years, including Ella's final days of confinement and passing. Another bed, one we had purchased in earlier years, became my nightly abode. And the weight of pain and loss seemed to palpably lessen. Next came the distribution of Ella's clothing, jewelry, rings and other personal adornments to close family members. This included a lifetime of treasured memorabilia, with their many emotional associations for each particular loved one. Certain emotionally sustaining items, such as a color chalk drawing in silhouette, I decided to keep. With these decisions and actions have come a lessening of the emotional pains that have bound me since that fateful day in September of 2000.

With the shedding of these closest and most emotionally binding possessions has come a lightening of mood and a clearing of the mind. Now, for the first time, I am aware of just how dark and dreary much of the house has become.... So I immediately pick up paint and brush and administer a coat of brightness to the kitchen and dining areas; then the same to the halls and utility room; and, most recently, the lightest of pastel mint green to the living room and bedroom. Everything is now twice as light as before. All of this is done in the midst of trying to solve the latest quandary: Shall I do all this and stay here with the memories of the last nine years? Or shall I do it all and make the move to smaller quarters? The decision to sell wins out, as I move further into the waters of bachelorhood.

In the midst of testing the waters and deciding to make the plunge, I am now feeling the rightness of the whole process! Now is the time! So I've just listed the house for sale and made an offer on a condominium. I don't know how it will turn out, but it just feels right. So, finally, I'm taking that leap of faith. And with that leap is coming the courage to part with other items common to Ella's and my life together, and bring into the home things reflecting **my** personal tastes – things like a brand new bedroom suite, and not too far in the future some new living room furniture and a dining room table. This year will probably also see the exchange of that thirteen-year-old 18" Sony TV and eleven-year old stereo system for a more modern and functionally integrated home entertainment center.

But other things representing our years of marriage will remain: The two chairs in the bedroom; the living room rocker, bought just after we were married; a ten-volume set of O. Henry books we inherited from Ella's parents; our silver, china and crystal; and a number of other things precious to our mutual memory.

After all of this is done and behind me, then, and only then, will I have taken the plunge and deeply immersed myself in the warming and freeing waters of my new life. Then will the parable have been fully acted out in **my** life. But, the testing will go on forever.

Transition: Is the Time Ripe?

February 15, 2002

When Ella died in September of 2000, a number of friends and professionals gave me these suggestions:

(1) Stay put for at least a year. Keep your living and financial arrangements stable while going through the early stages of grieving and healing.

(2) Don't make critical judgments on such things as when and how to dispose of your beloved's possessions. Don't make quick, and likely rash, decisions on what to give away and to whom.

(3) Give your heart and emotions a chance to experience the loss.

(4) Work through all the implications of what it will be like to be a "widow/widower". Learn to live with that new identity and its associated lifestyle.

(5) Let your feelings **and** thinking process bring you to the final decisions about all these vital decisions.

(6) Above all, find things to do and people to be with.

Well, it's easier said than done. I've taken

some suggestions to heart. But, it's been tough to follow a "cookbook recipe" for transitioning into a post-matrimonial status. I wrote extensively about decompressing and feeling a loss of identity when the caretaker role was gone; the constant heartache and episodic eruption into tears; and the load of depression that weighed over my very being. To others, I must have cut a pretty pathetic figure those first three or four months. I was really locked into that helping role, and all the accompanying attitudes.

However, along with the long-term venting of anger, grief and frustration, and with letting myself fully feel my loss came a springtime of the Soul, a renewal of energies, much like a new bud bursting forth from the stump of a freshly cut tree.... Interesting! My soul's spring-like renewal was coming even as the season of spring announced itself. As summer approached, my life energies continued to intensify. I was beginning to feel more and more like my pre-caregiver self. Then, things again began to slow down. Something about the grieving was incomplete. I finally decided it was that thing about Ella's ashes. They still sat in a box on her dresser, a daily reminder.

You know the rest of that story: My September 11th trip to the Outer Banks and a next day sunrise ceremony, committing my Beloved's ashes to the vast waters of the mighty Atlantic. My final release of Ella to God and my release of myself from her daily presence couldn't be completed by a rigid recipe. It came only by following an inner stirring of the soul to perform this final rite of passage – a symbol of her passage into the life of the Spirit, my releasing of myself back into this life of the flesh.

The proof that the timing was right, that my soul was ripe for this final event between us? Well, the "proof is in the pudding", as the old saw goes. Before September 12th, I couldn't part with many out-of-date and useless things if my life had depended on it. **Now**, in three months, I have literally "cleaned house". And with the removal of the many symbols of our daily life together has come a freeing of my emotions, to the point that I can now contemplate leaving "this old house" and moving on to new places and new events in my life.

Will I actually ever move? The future will tell. All I know now is that as the changes multiply by the day, my depression lifts and my spirit sings. Whether or not I will remarry, time will tell.

Was this the right time? For me, **yes it was**. How about others among you? You'll have to be the judge of that. I hope my story will help in your decision-making.

Yard Sale

March 17, 2002

Meine Frau, Ella, was a notorious shopper for secondhand merchandise. Whether it be plates, plaques, bells, books, or any other such treasure that struck her fancy, she was a lifelong patron of the once used, now unwanted trash of other folks. I learned early in our marriage that no yard/garage sale, flea market or antique dealer was exempt from her curiosity. And, furthermore, I quickly learned never to spurn Ella's quest for the unusual prize, often found in the seediest and most out-of-the-way places. No trip, whether a family visit or vacation jaunt, was ever completely satisfying to her unless it included a stroll through a flea market or a favorite "trash or treasures" outlet, consummated by a package or two clutched under her arm as we walked out, piled into the car, and resumed our journey.

So, not surprisingly, since my Beloved's death I have long surveyed the evidence of her lifelong passion for the banished goods of another, some things beautiful, others rather plain or even garish, by my standards: One-of-a-kind plates, over a hundred and fifty in number; a hundred and ten bells of varying sizes and types; fifty Teddy Bears from one inch in length to almost two feet; a number of vases and lamps; and books by the dozens, both esoteric and mundane. And most of these treasures remained in their sacredly designated places for over a year after Ella's passing. It was as if I had no vision, energy, or passion for breaking with familiar, yet haunting objects.

Yet, since the September 12th ritual of scattering my wife's ashes in the Atlantic, I have been in the middle of a frenetic race to clear out all of that "stuff". Just yesterday, I was up at 6:00 AM, setting up tables and placing the many already priced items in neat categories for the anticipated customers. Before my friend and Senior Center co-worker, Marisa, and I had completed the final setup at 6:45 AM, cars began streaming in. And before 8:00 AM, the official start of the sale, some two-dozen customers had arrived and departed with whatever they had deemed to be their prize-of-the-day. By 10:45 AM, the traffic had ceased and Marisa and I began returning the remaining unsold items to the safety of the house. Two-thirds of the smaller items left the premises. Three tables sold quickly. Those other larger items will have to go to family or charity.

An observation about my emotional state, while doing all the pricing of items the day before the yard sale: It was difficult to pick up an object and make a realistic assessment of what persons other than myself might pay for it. Looking at any number of objects with sentimental value, I found myself repeatedly thinking, "How can I put a monetary value on this thing that represents Ella's and my sharing for so many years?" It was most difficult, indeed. And, yet, as I watched each person pick up a particular item, handle it, size it up, I often saw a gleam in the eye that spoke of some hidden attraction, some desire to possess that object... for some unknown, unexamined reason. What I was having emotional pangs about parting with was at the same time finding a place in the mind and the heart of another. And my momentary grief at that particular loss softened, with the realization that someone else was now bestowing love on that "thing" that had once graced the Jeter household.

And that is how I am "down-sizing", how I am managing to divest myself of the things that once held a dear place in the hearts of two lovers, but now must go. Hanging on only kills the Spirit. Love is dynamic, ever changing. And I will find Love in new objects, new circumstances, perhaps even persons as yet unknown to me. That is my hope. That is my Faith.

A Lesson on Transformation

April 20, 2002

A most fascinating experience for me took place my first year on the farm – age eleven, to be more precise. All about us, the fields were turning green, and trees and shrubs were bursting forth with buds. All were harbingers of full foliage, flowering and eventual harvest time. But on one small branch of a sassafras tree there hung an object, a gray, dried mass, seemingly out of its proper time and place. On closer examination, it had very much the appearance of a miniature replica of a mummified pharaoh of ancient Egypt – a real puzzler, which I promptly showed to my mother.

"What you see looks dead, but inside there is the pupa of either a moth or butterfly." Discerning my questioning face, she explained the facts of life about the life and death of the adult moth/butterfly, and the surprising renewal of life for these beautiful aerial insects we would all see during the hot, short months of summer. Though Mother didn't say so in so many words, my child's mind eventually picked up the idea that something hidden was about to happen. Thereafter, almost daily, I managed to check out the dried shell that hid within it the "sleeping beauty" chrysalis of, I hoped, a butterfly.

A Lesson on Transformation

Then came the day that the dead-looking gray mass, suspended on its tiny rope of silken fibers, began shaking, as if pushed by some invisible force. I called Mother and my younger siblings to the spot, and we watched... and watched... and watched. Days came and went, and our apprehension sharpened, as the hidden pupa seemed to become larger, but remained encased in its silken tomb. All we children were concerned that the insect was going to tire itself out and die. "Shouldn't we cut a slit in the case and help it escape?" I naively asked. "No", Mother emphatically answered! "Our interfering with the chrysalis in its struggle may well interrupt its development into final form. Mother Nature's way is wisest. Let's just see what happens."

A few days later the dried case, now swollen, began to split wide open. We watched with wondering eyes as a winged creature began pushing out of its silk sarcophagus and grasped the sassafras twig with trembling feet. Within thirty minutes or so, the moth, now fanning its wings, dried out and took on a beautiful pale blue hue. In less than an hour, it had shed its stiff silken garment and taken to the air. The empty case that had so recently enclosed a sleeping pupa remained on the sassafras branch, its own silent witness to the wonderfully transforming event we children had also experienced.

This has become an up-to-date and personal lesson on the struggles necessary for one to leave the bonds of matrimony and embark on a new and different life-style: that of being single once more. The past six months seem analogous to the chrysalis struggling to leave its womb of silk and flex its newly formed wings: Preparing my home for sale was not without an emotional battle. It's a blessing that the home Ella and I had shared for her last seven years sold in ten days. I don't know how I would have fared, had the sales process drug out for many months, as is so typical in these difficult economic times. But it happened quickly, and my new place, a little condominium nest in New Kent Village, is rapidly taking on a personality that reflects my own personal tastes and new lifestyle. Significantly, all this recent activity has occurred in spring, the time when all of Life seems to find renewal, the time when great transformations of all kinds issue forth.

So, during these new days, like the freed chrysalis, **my** Spirit feels ever lighter and freer. My heart and my voice are singing with more joy and happiness; my feet are again feeling the energy and power of rhythm and dance; and, every so often, the clown or jokester in me rears its comedic head and tells me to not take things so seriously!

When I compare this state of being to the state of depression and anxiety I felt for the previous five or six years, I can come to no other conclusion: Before my very eyes, I am being freed. I am being emotionally changed from the hidden, struggling creature of so many years, to a being aware of God's Spirit, and free to move toward that Spirit.

So I feel blessed as never before. Out of the struggle, I have experienced **freedom,** and

joy, and **blessing.** That is the parable of the chrysalis. That is the Lesson of Transformation!

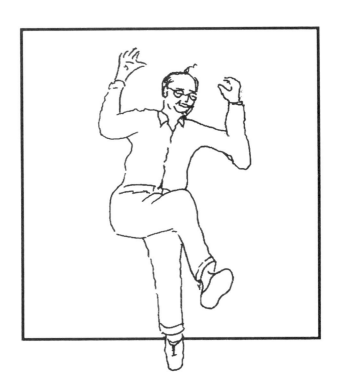

A Postscript on Bereavement

On Moving Beyond Adjustment

May 20, 2002

Yes, I'm now comfortably ensconced in my new condominium – for the past two months. And it feels like I'm awakening from a dream. I haven't felt this relaxed and at peace for many a year!

Several folks have asked, "How did you go through all the pressures, the trials and tribulations of caregiving, especially since Ella went under hospice care two years ago? You look so much better now than you did then." I have to confess that five years ago, right after her stroke, I lived in dread of all the possibilities that awaited both her in her disability, and me in my prospective responsibilities as the primary caregiver.

For many months now, I've written extensively of the multiple ministries provided my family by Rex Wellness Center, Resources for Seniors Total Life Center, Hospice of Wake County, and of course our loving daughter Alice and the many community and church friends. To this plethora of supportive folks I owe a debt of gratitude.

But enduring the caregiving load and the grief of loss goes far beyond mere "adjustment", for the sake of survival only. And this is where another, most beneficent person brought an added dimension to my personal recovery from

94

the loss of a lifetime mate: Dr. Kathi Middendorf, a social psychologist. I met her in June of 2000 while searching for a personal coach. I had begun a novel eighteen months before, with a gripping first scene. But, the idea and flow of word pictures had ceased abruptly – all during that period when Ella's condition had worsened rapidly. I was getting increasingly frustrated with this "failure", and depressed at the looming prospect of Ella's death.

Kathi Middendorf is a life coach, who focuses on the connection between mind, body and the spiritual dimension of human existence. She is also an interfaith minister, with a spiritual emphasis to her life coaching approach. More than a dozen years before, as a rehabilitation counselor, I had studied some of the early research on "psycho-neuro-immunology", a newly emerging scientific field which emphasizes human function as essentially a biological-psychological feedback system, all intimately connected by the body's all-encompassing neurological network. This was a big step beyond psychology's earlier concept of the mind being separate from the body. But, science still allowed no place for the spirit within a woman or a man. With my personal bent toward the spiritual, I was quickly drawn to Dr. Middendorf's approach.

In our very first session, Kathi put her finger on my basic problem: A lack of trust in my own nature as a human being, generally speaking. More specifically, she saw me as loaded with pessimism, depression and, key to it all, self-deprecation. I was convinced I didn't have what it took to write creatively, from within my own being. And I reinforced this constantly by telling myself that I couldn't do it!

I had already shared several Pot Pourri articles, a short story or two, and of course, that ill-fated first scene of the novel. Immediately, Dr. Middendorf's strategy was to bring me to an awareness of myself as unified in body, emotions, mind, and having an essentially **good** spiritual nature. She also reminded me that my long-term caregiving and imminent personal loss of Ella was taking its toll in my energy. It was natural to be depressed, blue and without creative energy, under such circumstances. Her comments: "You certainly can't expect to have your usual energy for writing, under these conditions. But I suspect that you also block your own energy by what you believe, and how you tell yourself that you **can't** do this or that. Look at what you've shown me! This is solid evidence that you **do** have what it takes to write – or to do anything else good in this life that you put your mind to."

"But, you have to talk to yourself, out of that faith, moment-by-moment, day-by-day. So, **relax**! Tonight, as you prepare for sleep, tell yourself that you **can** re-start that story. Visualize yourself writing, out of that inner flow, joyously and effortlessly – just as you did that first time you created a story, on demand and in twenty minutes. Tomorrow morning, get up and immediately act on the affirmation of the night before. If things don't improve quickly, keep it up, persistently. I'll bet your story will begin flowing again in a very short time. "

I took Kathi's suggestions to heart. The impulse to write again came upon me, and the story began to flow from my mind and on to the computer screen. By my next meeting with Dr. Middendorf, several new scenes had been fleshed out. Bi-weekly sessions with Kathi have proceeded with little interruption for almost two years. I now have almost four hundred pages of drama, action, dialogue, and still the story goes on!

Just as I could have accepted that I couldn't write any more on that story, so, in similar fashion, I could simply "adjust" to my new single life, as "the best I can do" and wait for the day I will die. But, I do believe there's still life in the Old Boy, and I'm very excited about what's still out there for me to explore – and to experience – and to enjoy.

Death , you'll just have to wait your turn!

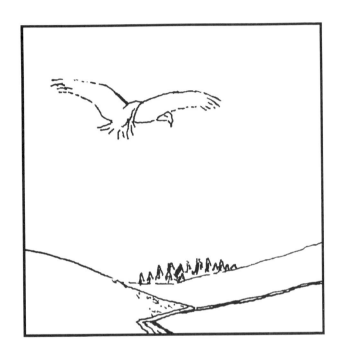

The ends of the earth are in thy
hands
The sea's dark deep and no man's
land
And I am thine, I rest in thee
Great Spirit, come, and rest in me.

The Lone Wild Bird, verse 2
Words by Henry Richard McFadyen.

Readers of *Walking Through the Valley* comment:

"I found the book to be excellent.... It's difficult to treat such a delicate subject with humor and sensitivity, and yet be objective.... With my parents, ages 88 and 89, now in a continuing care center, you have brought home to me the hope beyond the pain. This book should be recommended reading for all ministers, hospice workers, nursing and medical students, as well as be available to crisis and grief support groups." — Ilene Koenig, RN

"When I first met Bob, he was at the end of a fraying rope, close to breaking.... Thus began a series of weekly meetings, described in the book.... The first thing I did was urge him to seek out support from family, friends, and community. To his surprise, help came pouring in, beginning with his daughter, who continued to be a wonderful source of support throughout Ella's illness. The thing that struck me as I journeyed with Bob was his perseverance – his willingness to keep putting one foot in front of the other, confronting the obstacles along the path with a methodical stubbornness, refusing to yield to anything that was not in Ella's best interest. What also impressed me was his ability to bleed, to cry, to mourn, and finally to accept the long ending of her life. I belive that this book of essays offers a candid (and sometimes gritty) look at the day-to-day realities of caring for a long-suffering spouse. And Bob found ways to care for the caregiver, so that he could care for Ella. In so doing, he benefited them both" — Debie D. Saidla, PhD, Licensed Psychologist, Rex Healthcare

Order Form

Name: _____

Address: _____

_____

City, State, Zip: _____

Mail order form and check to:

Budding Bard Publishing

411 New Kent Pl

Cary, NC 27511-7603

For information call 919-380-9180

No telephone orders!

1-4 copies, $13.75 each

5 or more copies, $12.75 each

Please send the following:

_____ copies @ $13.75 = _____

_____ copies @ $12.75 = _____

Subtotal = _____

Sales tax (NC orders only) 6.5%_____

Shipping (US mail, 1st Class): $4.00 for first book, $1.50 for each additional book shipped to same address _____

TOTAL_____